MEAL
PLANNER

WEEKLY MEAL PLAN

WEEK OF:

	BREAKFAST	LUNCH	DINNER	SNACKS
SUNDAY				
MONDAY				
TUESDAY				
WEDNESDAY				
THURSDAY				
FRIDAY				
SATURDAY				

GROCERY LIST

MEAT

PRODUCE

DRY GOODS

REFRIGERATED

HOUSEHOLD

FROZEN

DELI/BAKERY

WEEKLY MEAL PLAN

WEEK OF:

	BREAKFAST	LUNCH	DINNER	SNACKS
SUNDAY				
MONDAY				
TUESDAY				
WEDNESDAY				
THURSDAY				
FRIDAY				
SATURDAY				

GROCERY LIST

MEAT

PRODUCE

DRY GOODS

REFRIGERATED

HOUSEHOLD

FROZEN

DELI/BAKERY

WEEKLY MEAL PLAN

WEEK OF:

	BREAKFAST	LUNCH	DINNER	SNACKS
SUNDAY				
MONDAY				
TUESDAY				
WEDNESDAY				
THURSDAY				
FRIDAY				
SATURDAY				

GROCERY LIST

MEAT

PRODUCE

DRY GOODS

REFRIGERATED

HOUSEHOLD

FROZEN

DELI/BAKERY

WEEKLY MEAL PLAN

WEEK OF:

	BREAKFAST	LUNCH	DINNER	SNACKS
SUNDAY				
MONDAY				
TUESDAY				
WEDNESDAY				
THURSDAY				
FRIDAY				
SATURDAY				

REFRIGERATOR INVENTORY

ITEM	QUANTITY	EXPIRATION

FREEZER INVENTORY

DISH	QUANTITY	ENJOY BY

PANTRY INVENTORY

ITEM	QUANTITY	EXPIRATION

GROCERY LIST

MEAT

PRODUCE

DRY GOODS

REFRIGERATED

HOUSEHOLD

FROZEN

DELI/BAKERY

WEEKLY MEAL PLAN

WEEK OF:

	BREAKFAST	LUNCH	DINNER	SNACKS
SUNDAY				
MONDAY				
TUESDAY				
WEDNESDAY				
THURSDAY				
FRIDAY				
SATURDAY				

GROCERY LIST

MEAT

PRODUCE

DRY GOODS

REFRIGERATED

HOUSEHOLD

FROZEN

DELI/BAKERY

WEEKLY MEAL PLAN

WEEK OF:

	BREAKFAST	LUNCH	DINNER	SNACKS
SUNDAY				
MONDAY				
TUESDAY				
WEDNESDAY				
THURSDAY				
FRIDAY				
SATURDAY				

GROCERY LIST

MEAT

PRODUCE

DRY GOODS

REFRIGERATED

HOUSEHOLD

FROZEN

DELI/BAKERY

WEEKLY MEAL PLAN

WEEK OF:

	BREAKFAST	LUNCH	DINNER	SNACKS
SUNDAY				
MONDAY				
TUESDAY				
WEDNESDAY				
THURSDAY				
FRIDAY				
SATURDAY				

GROCERY LIST

MEAT

PRODUCE

DRY GOODS

REFRIGERATED

HOUSEHOLD

FROZEN

DELI/BAKERY

WEEKLY MEAL PLAN

WEEK OF:

	BREAKFAST	LUNCH	DINNER	SNACKS
SUNDAY				
MONDAY				
TUESDAY				
WEDNESDAY				
THURSDAY				
FRIDAY				
SATURDAY				

REFRIGERATOR INVENTORY

ITEM	QUANTITY	EXPIRATION

FREEZER INVENTORY

DISH	QUANTITY	ENJOY BY

PANTRY INVENTORY

ITEM	QUANTITY	EXPIRATION

WEEKLY MEAL PLAN

WEEK OF:

	BREAKFAST	LUNCH	DINNER	SNACKS
SUNDAY				
MONDAY				
TUESDAY				
WEDNESDAY				
THURSDAY				
FRIDAY				
SATURDAY				

WEEKLY MEAL PLAN

WEEK OF:

	BREAKFAST	LUNCH	DINNER	SNACKS
SUNDAY				
MONDAY				
TUESDAY				
WEDNESDAY				
THURSDAY				
FRIDAY				
SATURDAY				

GROCERY LIST

MEAT

PRODUCE

DRY GOODS

REFRIGERATED

HOUSEHOLD

FROZEN

DELI/BAKERY

WEEKLY MEAL PLAN

WEEK OF:

	BREAKFAST	LUNCH	DINNER	SNACKS
SUNDAY				
MONDAY				
TUESDAY				
WEDNESDAY				
THURSDAY				
FRIDAY				
SATURDAY				

GROCERY LIST

MEAT

PRODUCE

DRY GOODS

REFRIGERATED

HOUSEHOLD

FROZEN

DELI/BAKERY

WEEKLY MEAL PLAN

WEEK OF:

	BREAKFAST	LUNCH	DINNER	SNACKS
SUNDAY				
MONDAY				
TUESDAY				
WEDNESDAY				
THURSDAY				
FRIDAY				
SATURDAY				

REFRIGERATOR INVENTORY

ITEM	QUANTITY	EXPIRATION

FREEZER INVENTORY

DISH	QUANTITY	ENJOY BY

PANTRY INVENTORY

ITEM	QUANTITY	EXPIRATION

GROCERY LIST

MEAT

PRODUCE

DRY GOODS

REFRIGERATED

HOUSEHOLD

FROZEN

DELI/BAKERY

WEEKLY MEAL PLAN

WEEK OF:

	BREAKFAST	LUNCH	DINNER	SNACKS
SUNDAY				
MONDAY				
TUESDAY				
WEDNESDAY				
THURSDAY				
FRIDAY				
SATURDAY				

GROCERY LIST

MEAT

PRODUCE

DRY GOODS

REFRIGERATED

HOUSEHOLD

FROZEN

DELI/BAKERY

WEEKLY MEAL PLAN

WEEK OF:

	BREAKFAST	LUNCH	DINNER	SNACKS
SUNDAY				
MONDAY				
TUESDAY				
WEDNESDAY				
THURSDAY				
FRIDAY				
SATURDAY				

GROCERY LIST

MEAT

PRODUCE

DRY GOODS

REFRIGERATED

HOUSEHOLD

FROZEN

DELI/BAKERY

WEEKLY MEAL PLAN

WEEK OF:

	BREAKFAST	LUNCH	DINNER	SNACKS
SUNDAY				
MONDAY				
TUESDAY				
WEDNESDAY				
THURSDAY				
FRIDAY				
SATURDAY				

GROCERY LIST

MEAT

PRODUCE

DRY GOODS

REFRIGERATED

HOUSEHOLD

FROZEN

DELI/BAKERY

WEEKLY MEAL PLAN

WEEK OF:

	BREAKFAST	LUNCH	DINNER	SNACKS
SUNDAY				
MONDAY				
TUESDAY				
WEDNESDAY				
THURSDAY				
FRIDAY				
SATURDAY				

REFRIGERATOR INVENTORY

ITEM	QUANTITY	EXPIRATION

FREEZER INVENTORY

DISH	QUANTITY	ENJOY BY

PANTRY INVENTORY

ITEM	QUANTITY	EXPIRATION

WEEKLY MEAL PLAN

WEEK OF:

	BREAKFAST	LUNCH	DINNER	SNACKS
SUNDAY				
MONDAY				
TUESDAY				
WEDNESDAY				
THURSDAY				
FRIDAY				
SATURDAY				

WEEKLY MEAL PLAN

WEEK OF:

	BREAKFAST	LUNCH	DINNER	SNACKS
SUNDAY				
MONDAY				
TUESDAY				
WEDNESDAY				
THURSDAY				
FRIDAY				
SATURDAY				

GROCERY LIST

MEAT

PRODUCE

DRY GOODS

REFRIGERATED

HOUSEHOLD

FROZEN

DELI/BAKERY

WEEKLY MEAL PLAN

WEEK OF:

	BREAKFAST	LUNCH	DINNER	SNACKS
SUNDAY				
MONDAY				
TUESDAY				
WEDNESDAY				
THURSDAY				
FRIDAY				
SATURDAY				

GROCERY LIST

MEAT

PRODUCE

DRY GOODS

REFRIGERATED

HOUSEHOLD

FROZEN

DELI/BAKERY

WEEKLY MEAL PLAN

WEEK OF:

	BREAKFAST	LUNCH	DINNER	SNACKS
SUNDAY				
MONDAY				
TUESDAY				
WEDNESDAY				
THURSDAY				
FRIDAY				
SATURDAY				

GROCERY LIST

MEAT

PRODUCE

DRY GOODS

REFRIGERATED

HOUSEHOLD

FROZEN

DELI/BAKERY

WEEKLY MEAL PLAN

WEEK OF:

	BREAKFAST	LUNCH	DINNER	SNACKS
SUNDAY				
MONDAY				
TUESDAY				
WEDNESDAY				
THURSDAY				
FRIDAY				
SATURDAY				

REFRIGERATOR INVENTORY

ITEM	QUANTITY	EXPIRATION

FREEZER INVENTORY

DISH	QUANTITY	ENJOY BY

PANTRY INVENTORY

ITEM	QUANTITY	EXPIRATION

FAVORITE BREAKFASTS

MEAL	COOKBOOK/WEBSITE

FAVORITE BREAKFASTS

MEAL	COOKBOOK/WEBSITE

FAVORITE LUNCHES

MEAL	COOKBOOK/WEBSITE

FAVORITE LUNCHES

MEAL	COOKBOOK/WEBSITE

FAVORITE DINNERS

MEAL	COOKBOOK/WEBSITE

FAVORITE DINNERS

MEAL	COOKBOOK/WEBSITE

Recipe:

Serving:

Prep Time:

Cook Time:

Temperature:

Ingredients:

Methods:

Wine Pairing:

From the Kitchen of:

Recipe:

Serving:

Prep Time:

Cook Time:

Temperature:

Ingredients:

Methods:

Wine Pairing:

From the Kitchen of:

Recipe:

Serving:

Prep Time:

Cook Time:

Temperature:

Ingredients:

Methods:

Wine Pairing:

From the Kitchen of:

Recipe:

Serving:

Prep Time:

Cook Time:

Temperature:

Ingredients:

Methods:

Wine Pairing:

From the Kitchen of:

Recipe:

Serving:

Prep Time:

Cook Time:

Temperature:

Ingredients:

Methods:

Wine Pairing:

From the Kitchen of:

Recipe:

Serving:

Prep Time:

Cook Time:

Temperature:

Ingredients:

Methods:

Wine Pairing:

From the Kitchen of:

Recipe:

Serving:

Prep Time:

Cook Time:

Temperature:

Ingredients:

Methods:

Wine Pairing:

From the Kitchen of:

Recipe:

Serving:

Prep Time:

Cook Time:

Temperature:

Ingredients:

Methods:

Wine Pairing:

From the Kitchen of:

Recipe:

Serving:

Prep Time:

Cook Time:

Temperature:

Ingredients:

Methods:

Wine Pairing:

From the Kitchen of:

Recipe:

Serving:

Prep Time:

Cook Time:

Temperature:

Ingredients:

Methods:

Wine Pairing:

From the Kitchen of:

Recipe:

Serving:

Prep Time:

Cook Time:

Temperature:

Ingredients:

Methods:

Wine Pairing:

From the Kitchen of:

Recipe: ______________________

Serving: ______________ Prep Time: ______________

Cook Time: ______________ Temperature: ______________

Ingredients:

Methods:

Wine Pairing: ______________________

From the Kitchen of: ______________________

Recipe:

Serving:

Prep Time:

Cook Time:

Temperature:

Ingredients:

Methods:

Wine Pairing:

From the Kitchen of:

Recipe:

Serving:

Prep Time:

Cook Time:

Temperature:

Ingredients:

Methods:

Wine Pairing:

From the Kitchen of:

Recipe:

Serving:

Prep Time:

Cook Time:

Temperature:

Ingredients:

Methods:

Wine Pairing:

From the Kitchen of:

Recipe:

Serving:

Prep Time:

Cook Time:

Temperature:

Ingredients:

Methods:

Wine Pairing:

From the Kitchen of:

www.ingramcontent.com/pod-product-compliance
Lightning Source LLC
Chambersburg PA
CBHW081557280526
45788CB00011B/3502
9781088552025